Distribution, publication, and copying in any form are prohibited and subject to damages.

TEN HYPNOSES

Copying, publishing, and sharing with third parties are only permitted with the written consent of the author. Please observe the notes on copyright and usage.

Distribution, publication, and copying in any form are prohibited and subject to damages.

Copying, publishing, and sharing with third parties are only permitted with the written consent of the author. Please observe the notes on copyright and usage.

Distribution, publication, and copying in any form are prohibited and subject to damages.

Ingo Michael Simon

TEN HYPNOSES

50
ANOREXIA

Copying, publishing, and sharing with third parties are only permitted with the written consent of the author. Please observe the notes on copyright and usage.

Distribution, publication, and copying in any form are prohibited and subject to damages.

© 2024 Ingo Michael Simon
All rights reserved.
Independently published
www.ingosimon.com

Important Notes for Urgent Attention:

The contents of this book are based on the practical experiences of the author with hypnosis applications and psychotherapy in a trance state. Although the author has strived for the utmost care, errors or misunderstandings in the presentation cannot be completely excluded. Therapeutic work with people and the application of hypnosis are solely the responsibility of the hypnotist. It cannot be ruled out that parts of this book may be misunderstood or that the application of a presented procedure may cause an undesirable reaction in the client. The author also assumes no co-responsibility if work with a client is carried out with reference to the statements in this book.

The Author:

Ingo Michael Simon studied psychology and education and is a hypnotherapist with practices in southwestern Germany and Switzerland. With the help of hypnosis-supported psychotherapy, he primarily treats people with persistent psychological conditions. His practice focuses on anxiety disorders, pathological compulsions, and psychosomatic illnesses. His therapeutic offerings mainly include classical and modern hypnosis applications and the dreamland therapy he developed himself.

Copying, publishing, and sharing with third parties are only permitted with the written consent of the author. Please observe the notes on copyright and usage.

Distribution, publication, and copying in any form are prohibited and subject to damages.

INTRODUCTION	6
COPYRIGHT AND USAGE	8
HYPNOSIS 1	10
HYPNOSIS 2	16
HYPNOSIS 3	24
HYPNOSIS 5	35
HYPNOSIS 6	40
HYPNOSIS 7	44
HYPNOSIS 8	51
HYPNOSIS 9	60
HYPNOSIS 10	67
ALL TITLES IN THE SERIES	73

Copying, publishing, and sharing with third parties are only permitted with the written consent of the author. Please observe the notes on copyright and usage.

Introduction

The series "Ten Hypnoses" is very well known in Germany, Austria, and Switzerland as a collection of texts for therapeutic work and is used by numerous psychotherapeutic practices, doctors, therapists, coaches, and other helping professionals. I am pleased to now be able to offer these texts in other countries as well.

Most therapists have their own methods for inducing and deepening trance as well as for exiting trance. Therefore, I have focused on the main part of the hypnosis. The texts in this book can be integrated as the main part into any hypnosis process. The texts in this collection use various hypnosis techniques. I will not explain these in detail, as I assume that users have the appropriate training. It is also not necessary to understand the exact structure or functioning of the different parts. The texts can simply be read aloud, and they will have their effect.

Decide for yourself which text best suits your client or patient at any given time. You can also combine passages from different texts. It is not about using all ten hypnoses in sequence. It is a selection of possibilities.

I want to emphasize that books cannot replace therapy. Psychotherapy or other therapeutic treatments involve much more. A careful diagnosis is the necessary basis for deciding on the use of methods, including whether hypnosis or one of my texts should be used. Even in this case, preparatory discussions, follow-up discussions during the session, and of course, a therapeutic concept for the sequence of sessions and the content approaches are essential parts of therapy. This cannot and should not be achieved with a collection of texts.

In any case, I wish you much success in your work and I am pleased if my text templates can contribute in a small way.

Ingo Michael Simon

Distribution, publication, and copying in any form are prohibited and subject to damages.

Copyright and Usage

Copying, publishing, and sharing with third parties is prohibited and only permitted with the written consent of the author. Please observe the following copyright and usage guidelines.

This work has been carefully crafted and created to the best of the author's knowledge and personal experience. It comprises text templates and application guidelines for professional hypnosis sessions. The author is a licensed psychotherapist with extensive experience in psychotherapy, coaching, and personal training using hypnotic techniques and methods. Nevertheless, the author and the publisher assume no liability for the accuracy of information, instructions, and advice, nor for any typographical errors. The author and publisher accept no responsibility or liability for the application of these texts and recommendations with clients or patients, nor for any potential consequences or unexpected reactions. It is expressly noted that the application of therapeutic and advisory techniques and formulations lies solely and entirely within the responsibility of the practitioner. This also applies to adherence to the

Copying, publishing, and sharing with third parties are only permitted with the written consent of the author. Please observe the notes on copyright and usage.

boundaries of legally regulated medical and therapeutic practices. The fact that a book containing action proposals is freely available for sale does not imply that its application with clients or patients is permitted for everyone.

Hypnosis 1

… … Anorexia has been with you for a long time, it has become a part of your daily life … … and of course, you've tried repeatedly to end it … … Perhaps sometimes you succeeded, or almost succeeded … … You kept thinking that you were too fat, always seeing yourself as much too big, but deep down, you always knew that wasn't true … … You had this deep feeling of not being good enough … … It was your belief that you weren't worth much … … probably because you experienced devaluation and abuse … … This could have been physical abuse or emotional exploitation and powerlessness … … When we feel powerless, we feel like we are beneath others and not as valuable … … Your mind knows that you are valuable, and it also knows that you weren't or aren't too fat … … You are far too thin, you know that … … And you want to change that, but you don't just want to gain weight … … You want to feel yourself again, to be able to accept yourself, and ideally, to love yourself as well … … But self-love is a big goal … … You will achieve it, but if it's easier, you can start with self-acceptance and then move to self-love in the next step ... ... So take the word self-love as the best form of affection you can give yourself right now ... ...

... ... When you look back and think about how you've dealt with your issue so far, you'll surely notice that you've often felt guilty ... ... Even when you might say you're not to blame for the anorexia ... ... Maybe your mind sometimes says that it just happened or that you had no control over it, and of course, you are not guilty ... ... But a part of you was often doubting ... ... a doubting voice was somehow in the background, asking if something was wrong with you or if you did something wrong that led to the anorexia ... ... Or you thought you should be stronger and just overcome all the difficulties that arose from it ... ... You've always been very hard on yourself ... ... And it's important to end that today ... ... to forgive yourself ... ... for all that you might have silently or even unconsciously blamed yourself for ... ... Imagine you embrace yourself inwardly, to tell yourself that you are good and that deep inside, everything is okay ... ... because deep inside, it's just you ... ... And with your gaze turned inward, you can simply rest and relax ... ... Now you don't have to achieve anything, overcome anything, let go of anything ... ... Just let the words you hear work for you ... ... That is enough ... ... Being here and listening, that is really enough ... ... [about 20 seconds of silence] ... ...

+++ Version 1: Anorexia, General +++

... ... Now you can feel the deep emotions or at least sense them, and over time, they will become clearer ... ... Of course, there are also painful and exhausting feelings, but the good thing about feelings is that they are never harmful ... ... What harms us is always our judgment of our feelings ... ... You have often rejected your feelings too, thinking you shouldn't feel the way you felt ... ... But the truth is that feelings are not under our control, and that's a good thing ... ... because when you feel your feelings, especially the painful ones, they will soon dissolve again ... ... because you learn from every feeling and then become free again ... ... In the end, the indestructible feeling of self-love remains, which always carries you ... ... and anorexia dissolves along with the pain ... ... Self-love brings you back to yourself ... ... and with that, to self-determination and self-awareness ... ... to health and strength ... ... and anorexia becomes unnecessary, becomes just a memory, nothing more ... ... You free yourself from anorexia on your path back to yourself ... ... You look forward to eating and being healthy again ... ... [about 20 seconds of silence] ... ...

+++ End of Version 1 +++

+++ Version 2: Anorexia, Relapse +++

... ... Now you can feel the deep emotions or at least sense them, and over time, they will become clearer ... ... Of course, there are also painful and exhausting feelings, but the good thing about feelings is that they are never harmful ... ... What harms us is always our judgment of our feelings ... ... And you feel guilt inside again ... ... guilt because the anorexia has returned ... ... You thought you had let it go and overcome it, but it came back ... ... There could be many reasons for that, but you are not guilty ... ... But accept the feeling of guilt and feel it, feel it deeply, because then you will also feel that there is another feeling behind it ... ... Maybe you can feel it or just sense it, but there are feelings behind the guilt ... ... So accept everything you feel now, because in doing so, you free these feelings, and then they will soon dissolve again ... ... because you learn from every feeling and then become free again ... ... In the end, the indestructible feeling of self-love remains, which always carries you ... ... and anorexia dissolves completely ... ... Self-love brings you back to yourself ... ... and with that, to self-determination and self-awareness ... ... to health and strength ... ... Anorexia dissolves completely ... ... [about 20 seconds of silence] ... ...

+++ End of Version 2 +++

... ... Now simply feel the calm and relaxation ... ... Now you are relaxed, while you think about your issue the whole time, thinking about anorexia the whole time ... ... That's how it's possible in trance ... ... You can look at and process the most difficult topics here and still be relaxed ... ... It can also be painful, and you may feel burdens, perhaps you've felt uncomfortable emotions, but that's completely okay, because you can also always feel relaxation again ... ... you can distance yourself from your issues much faster and therefore change things constructively ... ...

… … Exactly like you did today … … The time of anorexia is coming to an end and will soon be just a life experience, just a memory … … That takes time, and you're taking that time … … and every day, you are a little bit freer and more content … …

Hypnosis 2

Instructions for Execution

An anchor (or trigger) refers to a stimulus that is meant to evoke a certain feeling or thought. It acts as a signal perceived by the client that then triggers an internal process. The established anchor replaces the suggestion. In daily life, a client can use an anchor to initiate or create a desired state, even without a trance state. Many stimuli can be used as anchors/triggers. I work with the following possibilities, which I also use in the series "Ten Hypnoses":

- **Physical Anchors** (closing the hand, pressing the ball of the thumb ...)

- **Visual Anchors** (symbols, word cards ...)

- **Auditory Anchors** (signal sounds like phone rings, melodies ...)

- **Olfactory Anchors** (scented oils ...)

- **Tactile Anchors** (handheld objects, talismans ...)

I also differentiate between peri-hypnotic and post-hypnotic anchors. Peri-hypnotic anchors are those used primarily during hypnosis, where the therapist sets up the anchor and then repeatedly triggers it to complement suggestions and visualizations. Post-hypnotic anchors are set up mainly for use after the session, so the client can help themselves. Have a bottle of a pleasant scented oil ready. You must be able to open and close it. It should have a somewhat strong scent that the client does not already use. For example, if the client loves vanilla, then that scent is already strongly emotionally associated, as is perfume. It works best if it's a "new" scent that we suggestively charge with hypnosis. However, it doesn't have to be an unknown scent. It just shouldn't be one the client regularly uses.

+++ End of Instructions +++

…… Today we are working with a very special scent …… with a technique that makes it much easier for you to feel connected to yourself and thus let go of anorexia …… to accept yourself and forgive yourself for anything you have felt guilty about or still feel guilty about, because it is time for a new feeling of life in self-love and self-awareness and without anorexia ... ... It is time to accept yourself and learn from your decisions and actions ... ... You've already done this and continue to do so ... ... You understand and learn ... ... Now it's time to forgive yourself, to love yourself, and to let go of anorexia ... ... The scent of inner peace and self-love will today become an anchor for you ... ... whenever you smell it, you connect with yourself and accept yourself in peace and love and let go of everything related to anorexia ... ...

... [Have a bottle of a pleasant scented oil ready. You must be able to open and close it. It should have a somewhat strong scent that the client does not already use. For example, if the client loves vanilla, then that scent is already strongly emotionally associated, as is perfume. It works best if it's a "new" scent that we suggestively charge with hypnosis. However, it doesn't have to be an unknown scent. It just shouldn't be one the client regularly uses.] ...

... ... Now it's all about deep calm ... ... because in deep calm and relaxation, you are always very close to yourself ... ... you are always very close to your true feelings, because that's what's important ... ... Only close to yourself can you find inner peace and self-love … … And these feelings help you to let go of anorexia once and for all … … In deep calm and relaxation, you are in your healing center … … Today you reach the healing center through the calm of trance … … and in the future, you will reach your healing center with the help of the special scent that we associate with your healing center … … This scent, which you will perceive in a few moments, will become an anchor for you … … a tool of self-love … … You are now relaxing even deeper … … You can do it … … It's going very well for you … … You're just letting go … … You feel a deep and pleasant relaxation within you … … and you have the desire to go even deeper into this beautiful relaxation … … deeply relaxed … … relaxed in the center … …

… … Now, in this pleasant relaxation, you can meet yourself with serenity, let go of all criticism and self-accusation, and accept yourself … … You are now truly in your healing center … … You accept yourself in this moment … … The more clearly you can feel the relaxation now, the sooner you can let go of anorexia, because it has served its purpose … … So feel the relaxation and feel the healing self-love, you feel it deep within you, because it is there … …

Now ... ... Now it is succeeding for you ... ... You can feel peace and self-love ... ... and in self-love, you let go of anorexia ...

[Open the bottle and bring it to the client's nose] ... You are in your healing center ... [Remove and close the bottle] ... This is a special step ...

[Open the bottle and bring it to the client's nose] ... You are now in your healing center ... ... and you are letting go of anorexia now ... [Remove and close the bottle] ... Maybe you're already imagining how wonderful it will be when you can feel self-love again and also feel truly free ... ... over and over again ...

[Open the bottle and bring it to the client's nose] ... You can accept yourself ... [Remove and close the bottle] ... The healing center is within you ... [Open the bottle and bring it to the client's nose] ... The healing center within you ... [Remove and close the bottle] ...

... [The chosen scent has now become an anchor. Each further presentation of the scent reawakens or emphasizes this feeling. This way, the client can focus on their thoughts and wishes and repeatedly receive an impulse for relaxation and self-acceptance. As a peri-hypnotic anchor, the chosen scent can be used in subsequent sessions without needing to be re-established.] ...

+++ Version 1: Anorexia, General +++

... ... You think about anorexia again ... ... Recognize once more that it is really time to start eating healthily again and gain weight ...

[Open the bottle and bring it to the client's nose] ... Something has changed, because you can now accept yourself better ... [Remove and close the bottle] ... Often you have judged yourself and seen yourself as worthless ...

[Open the bottle and bring it to the client's nose] ... Now you know that you are valuable and lovable ... [Remove and close the bottle] ... and you know that life is worth living ... ...

[Open the bottle and bring it to the client's nose] ... You know that a healthy life is worth living ... ... You are on your way ... [Remove and close the bottle] ...

+++ End of Version 1 +++

+++ Version 2: Anorexia, Relapse +++

... ... You think about anorexia again ... ... You had ended it, but it came back once more ... ... You have used this return to find even more inner peace and to focus even more on self-love ... ... You recognize once more that it is exactly now time to start eating healthily again and gain weight ...

[Open the bottle and bring it to the client's nose] ... You can truly accept yourself now ... [Remove and close the bottle] ... No more self-reproaches ...

[Open the bottle and bring it to the client's nose] ... Now you know that you are valuable and lovable ... [Remove and close the bottle] ... and now you definitively choose a self-determined life without anorexia ... ...

[Open the bottle and bring it to the client's nose] ... Never again anorexia ... [Remove and close the bottle] ...

+++ End of Version 2 +++

It's really amazing how quickly you've managed to initiate an important change … … to reach and feel your healing center, the center of your emotions … … That's good … … You've learned that you can indeed find and experience closeness to yourself and your feelings … … and every time you inhale this scent … … when you can perceive it …

[Open the bottle and bring it to the client's nose]

… it reminds you that you can accept yourself and that you want to live a self-determined life, completely without anorexia …

[Remove and close the bottle] …

Hypnosis 3

... ... You want to end anorexia, you want to process the backgrounds and causes in the depths of your feelings and then let go of anorexia forever and return to a healthy life ... ... To do this, you now embark on an inner journey ... ... a journey into and through your imagination, because in your creative imagination, you can change your life ... ... you can achieve goals you thought were unreachable ... ... So let your imagination carry you and dream yourself to a faraway place ... ... far away and yet very close ... ... Enter the land of dreams, which you can shape and imagine for yourself ... ... The most beautiful land you know ... ... the most natural land you know ... ... the most beautiful nature, with mountains and valleys ... ... meadows and forests ... ... It unfolds before your inner eyes ... ... now ...

... ... Look around in your imagination ... ... You stand on a path that leads through the land of your dreams ... ... Perhaps through a blooming landscape ... ... or through a snowy landscape if you love winter ... ... It can be a summer day or a rainy autumn day, just as you wish ... ... It's your imagination, so it should be exactly how you like it best ... ... It should be so that you can feel comfortable ... ... So create the landscape yourself and follow the path ... ... Every path here is easy to walk, because every path in the land of dreams leads you to yourself ... ... You cannot get lost ... ... You walk step by step, and your thoughts go with you ... ... You think about anorexia, about the long journey you've already taken with it ... ... with all the highs and lows ... ... with the guilt and the feeling of being wrong ... ...

... ... You thought that you couldn't do anything right, couldn't do anything well enough, tried to find love and recognition ... ... and you kept trying to get a grip on your life, to be able to control it, but you felt powerless ... ... In the land of dreams, you are not powerless ... ... Everything here belongs to you alone, and you can decide everything for yourself here ... ... and you can also recognize ... ... recognize why things happened the way they did ... ... recognize that you can change things yourself and become healthy ... ... The path leads you to a special place ... ... it's a round place, and in the middle of this place lies a huge glass ball ... ... You walk very close and look inside, but it seems to be empty ... ... It feels smooth and cool, but then you suddenly notice that you can reach through the glass without breaking the ball ... ... You are in the land of dreams ... ... Nothing can be destroyed here, and nothing can break ... ... Here, there are no limits for you ... ... So you can also penetrate a glass ball ... ...

... ... So you take a big step into this ball and stand inside, and it is pleasantly warm ... ... You look out from inside, and then you gradually see images appearing on the glass wall ... ... like in a cinema or like a slide show, different images alternate, projected onto the inside of the ball ... ... Images of your own memories, images of your life ... ... maybe you see yourself in your daily life ... ... maybe pictures of your family or friends ... ... who knows, they appear on their own when you look ... ... and over time, you also recognize very special images ... ... images that show you how anorexia came about ... ... Perhaps there are just certain people that you suddenly recognize and who somehow contributed to anorexia ... ... perhaps some without even noticing, and perhaps there was one person or another whom you did not realize contributed to it ... ... Maybe you also see people who have often helped you ... ... Somehow everything and everyone we encounter in life contributes to our development, so all the people in your life contribute to your development ... ... and you also contribute to theirs ... ... But today, it's not about judgments, not about who made mistakes ... ... You probably have an assessment of that, but it's about something else, something much more important ... ... It's about the fact that deep inside, you once learned that anorexia was a way out ... ... not intentionally, not consciously, but you learned it that way ... ... It had to happen that way; you couldn't avoid it ... ... You would have needed help back then, but that help wasn't available ... ... Today, it is, because today you are in the land of your dreams, and today you learn anew and differently ... ...

+++ Version 1: Anorexia, General +++

... ... Today you learn on a much deeper and much stronger inner level ... ... You learn how to support yourself and accept yourself, yes, even love yourself ... ... even and especially when there is no one else who wants to or can love you ... ... And with that, you learn on a very deep level of your feelings how to see yourself as valuable and good, because that's what you are ... ... You now learn how to take care of your health and want to do so ... ... You now learn on a very deep level of your feelings to be close to yourself and to stay close to yourself ... ... Everything else falls into place because when you are close to yourself, you also recognize in your daily life that you should gain weight and that you can eat normal portions again ... ... Being close to yourself means accepting yourself and thus also loving yourself ... ... All of this you now learn as if by itself, deep inside ... ... The images inside make this constructive learning possible ... ... and anorexia dissolves within the ball ... ... [about 20 seconds of silence] ... ...

+++ End of Version 1 +++

+++ Version 2: Anorexia, Relapse +++

... ... Today you learn on a much deeper and much stronger inner level ... ... You learn how to support yourself and accept yourself, yes, even love yourself ... ... even and especially when you don't achieve your goals right away or when problems reappear ... ... You also learn that the return of anorexia was just a brief return, like a memory that you can let go of even faster ... ... So today, you learn especially to let go of anorexia once more … … You are getting closer and closer to yourself, and healthy eating, sufficient eating, and a healthy body weight are becoming more and more natural for you … … Let the images in the ball work for you … … Let your deepest inner self learn … … [about 20 seconds of silence] … …**+++ End of Version 2 +++**

… … Then you continue on … … Step by step … … and you think about how what you can experience so easily in your imagination can become reality … … Then you realize that it is already reality … … your new reality … … because the land of dreams is deep inside you … … It's always been there … … I'm just telling you about it … …

… … Now only your relaxation is important, your deep calm … … because it gently and safely leads you to true inner liberation … …

… … Now only your relaxation is important, your deep calm … … because it gently and safely leads you far away from anorexia … …

… … Now only your relaxation is important, your deep calm … … because it gently and safely directs all the words you hear into the depths of your emotions … …

… … Now only your relaxation is important, your deep calm … … because it gently and safely directs all the words to a helpful place deep inside … …

… … You now realign your thoughts completely … … and you think about the successes in your life … …

… … You now realign your thoughts completely … … and you think about previously achieved goals in your life … …

… … You now realign your thoughts completely … … and you draw confidence and hope from your thoughts and memories … …

… … You now realign your thoughts completely … … and your conviction and will to overcome anorexia grow stronger … …

… … Today you experience renewal, you experience the farewell to anorexia … …

… … Focus now on the conscious perception of your body feeling … … because in the feeling of your body, you recognize how you feel deep inside … …

… … Focus now on the conscious perception of your body feeling … … because with it, you also feel that it's about you, about your self-determination … …

… … Focus now on the conscious perception of your body feeling … … because with it, you also feel your great potential for renewal … …

… … Focus now on the conscious perception of your body feeling … … because with it, you feel exactly this great potential for true renewal … …

… … Today you experience renewal, you experience the farewell to anorexia … …

… … In your repertoire of feelings, there is always some self-love … … and now you can feel this feeling in you again … …

… … In your repertoire of feelings, there is always some self-love … … and now this feeling may fully enter your consciousness … …

… … In your repertoire of feelings, there is always some self-love … … and now this feeling may completely fill you … …

… … In your repertoire of feelings, there is always some self-love … … and this feeling helps you with healthy self-determination … …

… … Today you experience renewal, you experience the farewell to anorexia … …

+++ Version 1: Anorexia, General +++

… … You now choose a daily time for reflection … … because this makes it easy for you to focus on your healthy self-determination every day … …

… … You now choose a daily time for reflection … … because this way you experience self-love and self-awareness and self-determination every day as normal … …

… … You now choose a daily time for reflection … … because this way you can tap into your potential anew every day and use it for yourself … …

...... You now choose a daily time for reflection ...... because this way you say goodbye to anorexia and find your way back to self-love ......

...... Today you experience renewal, you experience the farewell to anorexia ......

+++ End of Version 1 +++

+++ Version 2: Anorexia, Relapse +++

...... You now repeat the already successful liberation from anorexia ...... because this way you remain permanently in healthy self-determination ......

...... You now repeat the already successful liberation from anorexia ...... because this way self-love and self-determination become normal once again and forever ......

...... You now repeat the already successful liberation from anorexia ...... because this way you can tap into your potential anew every day and use it for yourself ......

...... You now repeat the already successful liberation from anorexia ...... because this way you say goodbye to anorexia permanently and successfully ...... Now ......

… … Today you experience renewal, you experience the farewell to anorexia … …

+++ End of Version 2 +++

… … Now you feel the true and honest feeling of self-love and self-determination very intensely and consciously … … and you can feel this again and again in your everyday life … … This succeeds now, in this trance, and every coming day, and you will see that it is easy and completely natural to eat normally and healthily … …

… … Now you feel the true and honest feeling of self-love and self-determination very intensely and consciously … … and with that, the renewal really happens now and every day … … You have done it … … You have reached your goal … … You think and feel differently and anew … … You think and feel better, and you are sure that your self-love will grow even stronger … … Yes, you can do it … … Yes, you are doing it … … This is your success … … Yes, your success … …

Hypnosis 5

... ... You want to end anorexia once and for all ... ... Sometimes you succeeded, because there were phases when you actually ate normally and also had a normal weight ... ... It's possible to end this and build a healthy eating behavior permanently ... ... It's not really about food; it's more about self-determination when you starved yourself ... ... You had the impression that you no longer had control over your life, and then you decided that you could have this one power, to decide for yourself when and how much to eat ... ... and to not eat at all ... ... So it's about recognizing again that you can also control other areas of your life and that the recognition and love you missed cannot be forced by starving ... ... You can start by treating yourself lovingly ... ... Self-love is not everything, but it is the beginning of love and more than you've had so far ... ... So today, you walk the path of self-love ... ... Maybe that's too much, so you start with self-respect ... ...

... ... On this path, mindful attention to yourself helps ... ... the mindful treatment of yourself ... ... That sounds quite simple, and with the right approach, it is ... ... because in hypnosis, you can imagine many things more easily and create a good vision of a better future, of a very near future that begins today, in just a few moments ... ... with self-awareness and self-respect and also with affection and love from you for yourself ... ... for the end of anorexia, because only in self-love will it end ... ... What you need for this is a belief, an attitude of self-love that you can believe in, and you can believe in anything that you find as an honest attitude and conviction within you ... ... If you could look into an inner mirror and see a truth, a real conviction that would help you optimally on your path, then you could use this deep belief for yourself ... ... for the beginning of true self-love and for the end of anorexia ... ... and exactly this look into an inner mirror is possible today ... ... In this hypnosis, that is possible ... ... Now ... ...

... ... So now look into your inner mirror and discover a deep attitude there ... ... Look at yourself in this mirror, in the healthiest attitude you can imagine, and then you will see a writing that shows your deep attitude, because there is an important belief written there ... ... It says ... {5-10 seconds of pause} ...

+++ Version 1: Anorexia, General +++

... ... I embrace myself in love and protect myself today and every day with my mindfulness ... ...

+++ End of Version 1 +++

+++ Version 2: Anorexia, Relapse +++

... ... I know that I can love myself, and that's why I am worth letting go of anorexia once and for all ... ...

+++ End of Version 2 +++

... ... And now this attitude works noticeably and healingly for you ... ... The words you have heard correspond to your deep attitude and your own truth ... ... They become an affirmation that you can consciously and actively use by thinking or speaking them and reaffirming them again and again ... ... For self-love and healthy eating behavior, these words, this affirmation of healing and self-love, may now work deeply within you with your permission ... ... and take a firm place within you ... ... as a firm and stable belief ... ... as the foundation of your new emotionality ... ... for self-love and self-awareness ... ... for eating with pleasure and moderation ... ... for a new and good feeling of life, completely without anorexia ... ...

... ... Let these healing words work for you once more so that your self-awareness and self-love become even stronger ... ... Step by step stronger, because you need them more than anything else, more than anorexia ... ... Say it once more inwardly or read it from the inner mirror ... ...

+++ Version 1: Anorexia, General +++

... ... I embrace myself in love and protect myself today and every day with my mindfulness ... ...

+++ End of Version 1 +++

+++ Version 2: Anorexia, Relapse +++

... ... I know that I can love myself, and that's why I am worth letting go of anorexia once and for all ... ...

+++ End of Version 2 +++

… … Now let these words work and let them be there … … Allow these words to unfold their healing effect … … their liberating effect … … Now … …

… … In this hypnosis, words of self-respect and affirmations become healing beliefs when they help you on your way, when they correspond to your desire … … above all, when they are shaped by self-respect and turning towards yourself … … Your goal is to free yourself from anorexia, once and for all, and thus a return to self-respect and self-love … … and for that, you have read your affirmation and adopted it as a thought … … that's why it has already become your conviction … … And whenever you consciously and deliberately speak or think your affirmation, you lovingly support yourself on your way … … just like today … … just like here and today … …

Hypnosis 6

… … While you can feel the surface that supports your body well and feel that you are lying/sitting securely and stably, you can still feel into your surroundings with your senses and hear and understand my words well … … and you feel the loving and honest connection to yourself … …

… … You can move your arms and legs if you want and of course also feel that you can change your position if you want to be more comfortable. You can make all these decisions yourself … … and you can also decide about the end of anorexia, because you have the right and the power to end anorexia … …

… … You can calmly follow my words in your thoughts and either reject them or accept them … … And so, you can also reject anorexia, lovingly turn towards yourself, and find new ways of liberation … …

+++ Version 1: Anorexia, General +++

... ... You can still hear the sounds of your surroundings if you want, but you can also ignore them if you want to have peace and quiet, and you can bring the words that interest you to the forefront or simply wait and see how it happens naturally, just as you want ... ... and you naturally recognize self-love within you again ... ...

... ... Any significant change in your surroundings would immediately catch your attention, and you would certainly notice if my words speak of changes. With a little attention, you would also feel the effect of my words ... ... So, you also feel the clear change within you, that you can accept and love yourself ...

... ... You can direct and focus your attention independently. You can perceive the outside world or more of the inside, just as you wish ... ... and more and more, you recognize that you are worth saving yourself and that you are worth treating yourself with dignity, and therefore, you also decide to end anorexia ... ...

+++ End of Version 1 +++

+++ Version 2: Anorexia, Relapse +++

...... You can still hear the sounds of your surroundings if you want, but you can also ignore them if you want to have peace and quiet, and you can bring the words that interest you to the forefront or simply wait and see how it happens naturally, just as you want ...... and you immediately recognize self-love within you again ......

...... Any significant change in your surroundings would immediately catch your attention, and you would certainly notice if my words speak of changes. With a little attention, you would also feel the effect of my words ...... So, you feel that you want to end anorexia once and for all, because you have already succeeded in doing so once, so also today ......

...... You can direct and focus your attention independently. You can perceive the outside world or more of the inside, just as you wish ...... and you remember that you want and can save yourself because you insist on treating yourself with dignity, and therefore you end anorexia once and for all ...... Now ......

+++ End of Version 2 +++

... ... You can now completely surrender to calmness and comfort if you want, and even relax so deeply that you sink into a beautiful dream as if you were sleeping if you have the desire to dream, and once your optimal state of rest has set in and you feel that you are optimally relaxed, you can enjoy it even more ... ... and rejoice in your rediscovered self-love, because self-love ends anorexia and brings you back to a healthy and constructive life ... ... These are your feelings ... ... This is your path ... ... your path of saving your life ... ...

Hypnosis 7

... ... Today, you want to achieve something important ... ... You want to end anorexia and reestablish healthy eating habits ... ... You can achieve this goal today ... ... It only requires taking a clear position by focusing completely inwardly on your self-declared and honest intention ... ... Now, that's possible because you are in trance ... ... Now, it's happening just as you want it to ... ... Become aware of the outer world and then just as consciously turn inward ... ... It's very easy ... ... Just follow my words that guide and lead you ... ...

... You feel the surface that supports your body ... [about 5 seconds of pause] ...

... You recognize that you are lying/sitting securely and stably ... [about 5 seconds of pause] ...

... With your senses, you can still feel your surroundings ... [about 5 seconds of pause] ...

... You hear and understand all my words well ... [about 5 seconds of pause] ...

... And you feel this loving and honest connection to yourself ... [about 5 seconds of pause] ...

... You can move your arms and legs if you want ... [about 5 seconds of pause] ...

... You can change your position if it should be more comfortable ... [about 5 seconds of pause] ...

... You make all decisions yourself ... [about 5 seconds of pause] ...

... You can also decide for yourself about the end of anorexia ... [about 5 seconds of pause] ...

... Only you have the power over anorexia and its end ... [about 5 seconds of pause] ...

... You can calmly follow my words in your thoughts ... [about 5 seconds of pause] ...

... You can reject my words or accept them ... [about 5 seconds of pause] ...

... And so, you reject anorexia today ... [about 5 seconds of pause] ...

... So, you turn towards yourself today ... [about 5 seconds of pause] ...

... And you find your way to freedom from anorexia ... [about 5 seconds of pause] ...

+++ Version 1: Anorexia, General +++

... You can hear the sounds of your surroundings if you want ... [about 5 seconds of pause] ...

... You can also ignore the sounds ... [about 5 seconds of pause] ...

... Let the words that interest you come to the forefront ... [about 5 seconds of pause] ...

... Or just wait and see how it happens naturally ... [about 5 seconds of pause] ...

... And naturally, you recognize self-love deep within you ... [about 5 seconds of pause] ...

... Any significant change in your surroundings would immediately catch your attention ... [about 5 seconds of pause]

... You would certainly notice if my words speak of changes ... [about 5 seconds of pause] ...

... With a little attention, you would also feel the effect of my words ... [about 5 seconds of pause] ...

... So, you also feel the clear change within you ... [about 5 seconds of pause] ...

... And you feel that you want and can love yourself ... [about 5 seconds of pause] ...

... You can direct and focus your attention independently ... [about 5 seconds of pause] ...

... You can perceive the outside world or the inside, just as you wish ... [about 5 seconds of pause]

... And inwardly, you walk the path of saving your life ... [about 5 seconds of pause] ...

... You walk the path of dignity and protection of your body ... [about 5 seconds of pause] ...

... You walk the path of freedom from anorexia ... [about 5 seconds of pause] ...

+++ End of Version 1 +++

+++ Version 2: Anorexia, Relapse +++

... You can hear the sounds of your surroundings if you want ... [about 5 seconds of pause] ...

... You can also ignore the sounds ... [about 5 seconds of pause] ...

... Let the words that interest you come to the forefront ... [about 5 seconds of pause] ...

... Or just wait and see how it happens naturally ... [about 5 seconds of pause] ...

... And immediately, you recognize the familiar self-love deep within you ... [about 5 seconds of pause] ...

... Any significant change in your surroundings would immediately catch your attention ... [about 5 seconds of pause]

... You would certainly notice if my words speak of changes ... [about 5 seconds of pause] ...

... With a little attention, you would also feel the effect of my words ... [about 5 seconds of pause] ...

... You feel that it is time to end anorexia once and for all ... [about 5 seconds of pause]

... You have already succeeded once, so especially today ... [about 5 seconds of pause] ...

... You can direct and focus your attention independently ... [about 5 seconds of pause] ...

... You can perceive the outside world or the inside, just as you wish ... [about 5 seconds of pause]

... You want and can save yourself forever ... [about 5 seconds of pause] ...

... You want and can experience dignity and protection ... [about 5 seconds of pause] ...

... You want and can stop anorexia once and for all ... Now ... [about 5 seconds of pause] ...

+++ End of Version 2 +++

... You can now completely surrender to calmness and comfort ... [about 5 seconds of pause] ...

... You can now dream beautifully as if you were asleep ... [about 5 seconds of pause] ...

... And you can enjoy the depth of sleep and dreaming ... [about 5 seconds of pause] ...

... Above all, you rejoice in the rediscovered self-love ... [about 5 seconds of pause] ...

... This self-love ends anorexia ... [about 5 seconds of pause] ...

... Now begins a new and healthy time ... [about 5 seconds of pause] ...

Hypnosis 8

Instructions for Execution

The following hypnosis texts are structured so that they can be done as "normal" hypnosis or as self-hypnosis training. If you want to teach your client how to do effective self-hypnosis at home with this hypnosis, also read the sections {Only for Self-Hypnosis Training}, which you can otherwise omit and still have a good hypnosis session for your practice. A self-hypnosis trigger is a signal (action, image, or perception) that initiates the state of trance. With its help, even an inexperienced client can continue working with self-hypnosis at home. Of course, they can "only" work with simple suggestions that they can remember well and that we should prepare, or also with simple visualizations. Triggered self-hypnosis is a very good tool to give the client a task to continue therapy between sessions. A completely self-directed self-hypnosis, without a trigger, is also easy to learn, but it takes a lot of time and practice. Setting up the trigger is a fairly simple task and, of course, relieves the client, as I don't want to burden them with practicing a self-directed self-hypnosis. Contrary to all naysayers, I also claim here that it is really not a problem to teach a client simple trigger self-hypnosis. It is no more dangerous than meditation, autogenic training, or yoga. People survive these at home too. I have seen many patients in my practice who not only managed self-hypnosis well but enjoyed it. And when a patient enjoys doing self-hypnosis, no matter how simple the suggestion in the main part may look, it is a very good support for compliance.

+++ End of Instructions +++

… … Today you can free yourself from anorexia, you can finally stop starving and get healthy … … You have realized and understood that anorexia took control when you felt particularly powerless … … But in the meantime, you have regained control over your life, regained self-determination … … So it's time to end anorexia … … You will do that today, you will succeed with this hypnosis … … learn on a very deep level how to do it as quickly as possible … … {Only for Self-Hypnosis Training: … You can even learn how to do this hypnosis yourself because that's easy too … I'll show you how to do it, and as if by itself, your subconscious mind will learn in today's hypnosis how you can do self-hypnosis very quickly and reliably ... anytime and wherever you want ...} ...

... ... First of all, it's about getting into a very deep relaxation now with a simple thought or a simple trick, into a state where you can best reach the very deep level of change ... ... Once you've arrived there, you'll ensure real change ... ... for the end of anorexia because you gain even more self-determination and control over your life ... ... That succeeds today ... ... Imagine a balloon that is very light and carried by the wind ... ... flying higher and higher, and with it, your thoughts fly above the clouds ... ... Imagine the balloon flying before your inner eye, and you feel inner peace because your thoughts fly with it ... [5 seconds of pause] ... That's enough ... ... {Only for Self-Hypnosis Training: ... And the best part is that with this image, you can go into trance at home too, because you have done it now ... ... Whenever you close your eyes to find deep and liberating peace, and imagine a balloon flying above the clouds, you go immediately into a pleasant and comfortable trance ... just like now ... simply close your eyes, breathe calmly, and then let the balloon rise and keep your focus on this image, on this idea, until you become quite sleepy ...} ...

... ... You want to end the eating disorder, to end anorexia today ... ... Maybe you have a specific reason for starving ... ... perhaps you know why you do it ... ... or you can't exactly say why and how it came about ... ... But you know it was a form of taking control because you felt so powerless ... ... Today, you gain control through self-confidence and self-determination ... ... Then you no longer need to starve ... ... But first, relax even deeper, then it will be even easier to truly become free ... ... Imagine you are relaxing over ten simple steps and say ... ... I am going deeper now once ... ... I am going deeper now twice ... ... I am going deeper now three times ... ... I am going deeper now four times ... ... I am going deeper now five times ... ... I am going deeper now six times ... ... I am going deeper now seven times ... ... I am going deeper now eight times ... ... I am going deeper now nine times ... ... I am going deeper now ten times ... ... and then you are very, very deep in trance, but you can control everything yourself ... ... Now ... ... {Only for Self-Hypnosis Training: ... exactly like this, you deepen your trance at home, in your self-hypnosis, simply by inwardly going deeper step by step and counting, just as you have just heard ... and you will recognize and experience that you can relax deeply and talk to yourself at the same time ... You can simply whisper the words of relaxation and relax while keeping full control ... very easily and very safely ...} ...

+++ Version 1: Anorexia, General +++

... ... Now, in the pleasant relaxation ... ... in the depth of your thoughts and feelings, you can really free yourself from anorexia, every day anew, if you want ... ... End anorexia now by actively and consciously thinking ... ... I am self-confident and strong once, and I am eating again ... ... I am self-confident and strong twice, and I am eating again ... ... I am self-confident and strong three times, and I am eating again ... ... I am self-confident and strong four times, and I am eating again ... ... I am self-confident and strong five times, and I am eating again ... ... I am self-confident and strong six times, and I am eating again ... ... I am self-confident and strong seven times, and I am eating again ... ... I am self-confident and strong eight times, and I am eating again ... ... I am self-confident and strong nine times, and I am eating again ... ... I am self-confident and strong ten times, and I am eating again ... ... And then anorexia is over ... ... You are free again ... ...

{Only for Self-Hypnosis Training: ... And when you bring yourself into trance and have deepened it, you can whisper this suggestion to yourself ... just as you heard it here and today by whispering ten times ... ... I am self-confident and strong once, and I am eating again ... ... twice ... three times ... ... and so on until you say ... ... I am self-confident and strong ten times, and I am eating again ... ... That's how easy it is, and you can do it yourself ...} ... Now enjoy this new feeling of life ... ... Feel that you are completely self-determined and self-confident in your thoughts ... ... Feel that you have become free in your feelings ... ... Nothing can stop you ... ... because you have decided for yourself ... ... You are free ... ... You are truly free ... ... [About 20 seconds of silence] ...

+++ End of Version 1 +++

+++ Version 2: Anorexia, Relapse +++

... ... Now, in the pleasant relaxation ... ... in the depth of your thoughts and feelings, you can free yourself from anorexia once again; you know that it works because you have already succeeded ... ... So end anorexia now once and for all by actively and consciously thinking ... ... I am self-confident and once stronger than anorexia ... ... I am self-confident and twice stronger than anorexia ... ... I am self-confident and three times stronger than anorexia ... ... I am self-confident and four times stronger than anorexia ... ... I am self-confident and five times stronger than anorexia ... ... I am self-confident and six times stronger than anorexia ... ... I am self-confident and seven times stronger than anorexia ... ... I am self-confident and eight times stronger than anorexia ... ... I am self-confident and nine times stronger than anorexia ... ... I am self-confident and ten times stronger than anorexia ... ... And then anorexia is over ... ... You are free again ... ...

{Only for Self-Hypnosis Training: ... And when you bring yourself into trance and have deepened it, you can whisper this suggestion to yourself ... just as you heard it here and today by whispering ten times ... ... I am self-confident and once stronger than anorexia ... ... twice ... three times ... ...

and so on until you say ... ... I am self-confident and ten times stronger than anorexia ... ... That's how easy it is, and you can do it yourself ...} ... Now enjoy this new feeling of life ... ... Feel that you are completely self-determined and self-confident in your thoughts ... ... Feel that you have become free in your feelings ... ... Nothing can stop you ... ... because you have decided for yourself ... ... You are free ... ... You are truly free ... ... [About 20 seconds of silence] ...

+++ End of Version 2 +++

... ... {Only for Self-Hypnosis Training} ... ... When you do self-hypnosis at home, proceed exactly as you have experienced here ... ... It is completely simple and safe ... ... Start with the image of the rising balloon and imagine it until you feel that you are coming to rest ... ... Then whisper the suggestion to yourself ... ... I am going deeper now once, twice, and so on until you say: I am going deeper now ten times ... ... Then whisper your special suggestion ten times ... [Repeat the main part suggestion here] ... ... Then you may rest, and to wake up, imagine standing in freezing rain and then simply say: I am waking up again - One - Two -

Three ... ... Then you can open your eyes and be awake ... ... It's really that simple ... ... It works for you just like here and today ... ... You go into trance, free yourself, and wake up very simply again ... ...

Hypnosis 9

Instructions for Execution

Ideomotor activity refers to the phenomenon that our body follows our feelings and thoughts with movements. In everyday life, this following is shown as body posture, muscle tension, and movement patterns of a person, which naturally change with the mood and thoughts. In trance, ideomotor signals can be used to receive information that the client cannot actively communicate. The subconscious can, for example, answer questions with an agreed finger signal. Of course, ideomotor reactions can also be used suggestively, for example, with arm levitation and catalepsy. Ideomotor activity strengthens the trust in hypnosis and in one's ability to change and thus promotes therapy.

+++ End of Instructions +++

… … You are determined to end anorexia … … You know that it's good to do things well and carefully … … You also know that you don't have to be perfect for that … … no one has to be, because success does not lie in perfection ... ... You have often tried to be perfect, focused on performance, on performance and control ... ... until you finally controlled your eating so much that you almost starved ... ... You believed that you were too fat ... ... tried to be perfect and function perfectly ... ... and above all, you wanted to decide for yourself and have power over your life ... ... All of this you can use today to free yourself from anorexia because you have recognized that it would kill you ... ... Today, you can and may take control ... ... control over anorexia, and with your control, you end it today ... ... Your subconscious helps you because in this special trance, in your hypnosis today, that is possible ... ... In trance, you have more power and more freedom than ever before ... ... and the best part is that you don't have to wait to see if it works ... ... You can check it right away because your subconscious gives you a reliable sign of success in letting go ... ... for your success in letting go of anorexia ... ... Your subconscious can show you directly that it has achieved this with you ... ... Maybe you're already looking forward to it and are curious about how your subconscious will give you this sign ... ... and you can be sure that it will do so ... ... Then anorexia disappears ... ... So, let's go ...

... ... Imagine now how free you will be once you feel comfortable in your life again ... ... able to control your life and stay healthy ... ... how good it can feel to eat normally and take care of your health even in the face of failures and disappointments ... ... Now lay both hands loosely beside your body ... ... Now it's just your subconscious that is required ... ... You couldn't end anorexia before because you didn't see any other way to live a self-determined life ... ... But now it's much easier because now your subconscious can finally do it for you ... ... with your permission, because that's all that's required now ... ... My words now flow directly into your subconscious and help you with your liberation ... ... Your subconscious frees you from anorexia and immediately replaces it with self-confidence and self-assurance ... ... The perfect goal, the perfect request you send to your subconscious now is ... ... Free me from anorexia and give me self-confidence ... ... well done ... ... This request is the starting signal for your subconscious to begin your liberation now ... ... and already the tormenting perfectionism, all disappointments and hurts, and everything that contributed to anorexia flow into your right hand ... ... All inner burdens and all emotional pain you have experienced flow into your right hand and make it heavy ... ... All burdens gather in your right hand ... ... well done ... ... You can do it ... ... You're doing it right ... ... Only your right hand holds the inner burdens ... ... and now you can free yourself from them because deep inside, everything has already been resolved ... ... The last part of letting go can now be done by your body ... ... Your right hand holds all the burdens and all the disappointments ... ... So your hand can now let go of them forever ... ... That's how you become free and light inside ... ... and free yourself from anorexia ... ...

... ... Your subconscious has already successfully let go ... ... and now your body lets go too, and you can observe and clearly feel how the tormenting anorexia really falls away from you ... ... forever ... ... because your right hand now becomes very light, very light ... ... and because your hand becomes so light, it rises upwards, as if pulled by an invisible force, and then places itself on your stomach, on your solar plexus ... ... Your subconscious does this for you ... ... It moves your hand as if by itself and places it on your solar plexus ... ... as confirmation of your liberation and as a sign of your connection with yourself, as a sign of your self-confidence ... ...

+++ Version 1: Anorexia, General +++

... ... The more you succeed in letting go of anorexia now forever and at the same time building self-confidence, the more your right hand rises upwards ... ... You may already feel it, already feel how light your right hand becomes ... ... It rises upwards, feather-light and all by itself, because your subconscious does this for you ... ... Your subconscious now lifts your right hand and moves it slowly over your body and finally places it on your solar plexus ... ... and as soon as that happens, you know that anorexia is over, because that's the only reason your subconscious does all this ... ... It only makes sense if anorexia really comes to an end ... ... So, feel your right arm and your hand, it rises and moves over your body and places itself on your solar plexus ... ... for the end of anorexia ... ... It succeeds ... ... [Wait until the hand is really on the client's stomach! Stay with further suggestions until this has occurred!] ...

+++ End of Version 1 +++

+++ Version 2: Anorexia, Relapse +++

… … Today you process everything that has not yet succeeded and therefore end anorexia once and for all … … the more this final end of anorexia is really decided this time, the more your right hand rises upwards … … You feel it exactly … … It rises upwards because anorexia is ending … … Your subconscious now lifts your right hand and moves it slowly over your body and finally places it on your solar plexus … … and as soon as that happens, you know that anorexia is now finally and completely over, because that's the only reason your subconscious does all this … … It only makes sense if anorexia really comes to an end … … So, feel your right arm and your hand, it rises and moves over your body and places itself on your solar plexus … … for the final end of anorexia … … It succeeds now … … [Wait until the hand is really on the client's stomach! Stay with further suggestions until this has occurred!] …

+++ End of Version 2 +++

… … Well done … … very well done … … Now everything is different … … You have let go of anorexia and are full of self-confidence, and you are free … … Your subconscious now hands back full control of your hands, which feel good … … You can check it … … Move your hands and fingers and feel that your hands are completely under your conscious control … … well done … … It's time … … A new part of your life begins right now … … You have successfully let go of anorexia today … … and above all … … You were able to check for yourself that it really succeeded because it was agreed with your subconscious that it would place your hand on your body as a sign of success … … So, you have achieved your goal … …

Hypnosis 10

… … You know it well … the feeling of powerlessness and loneliness and the constant hunger … … You have experienced exactly that … The hunger was the only thing you could decide for yourself, without others taking control of your life … … But you have also tried to get out of it … … Sometimes you may have succeeded, but then the feeling of powerlessness and helplessness returned … … and you suddenly felt too fat, could no longer recognize yourself … … But you have also partially and repeatedly managed to free yourself and walk new paths … … So, today too … … Today, you achieve real liberation and real renewal … … Today, I achieve lasting liberation … … Today, I achieve lasting renewal … … and then a new feeling of self-determination and freedom arises … … For this, you meet yourself, now go deep into your feeling … … deeper than usual … … Today, your gaze turns completely inward, and with your gaze, your thoughts go inward … … and with your thoughts, your feelings go inward … … because there is real self-love … …

deep inside you ... ... and self-love is the key to any change ... ... So, lovingly speak to yourself and say ... ...

... ... I accept the time of anorexia and also the time of change ... ... because only I can and may determine that ... ...

... ... {about 5-10 seconds of silence} ...

... ... I accept the time of anorexia and also the time of change ... ... because only I can and may process my story and grow from it ... ...

... ... {about 5-10 seconds of silence} ...

... ... I accept the time of anorexia and also the time of change ... ... because only I can and may let go of anorexia right now and be free ... ...

... ... {about 5-10 seconds of silence} ...

... ... I accept the time of anorexia and also the time of change ... ... because only I can now create a new feeling of life ... ...

... ... {about 5-10 seconds of silence} ...

… … I accept the time of anorexia and also the time of change … … because only I am now at the center of my thoughts and feelings … …

… … {about 5-10 seconds of silence} …

+++ Version 1: Anorexia, General +++

… … I forgive myself for starving myself for so long … … because I am now truly ready to let go of guilt … …

… … {about 5-10 seconds of silence} …

… … I forgive myself for starving myself for so long … … because I am now truly ready to end the past … …

… … {about 5-10 seconds of silence} …

… … I forgive myself for starving myself for so long … … because I am now truly ready to look and move forward … …

… … {about 5-10 seconds of silence} …

… … I forgive myself for starving myself for so long … … because I am now truly ready to accept myself fully … …

… … {about 5-10 seconds of silence} …

… … I forgive myself for starving myself for so long … … because I am now truly ready to be myself … …

… … {about 5-10 seconds of silence} …

+++ End of Version 1 +++

+++ Version 2: Anorexia, Relapse +++

… … I forgive myself for slipping back into anorexia … … because I am now truly ready to let go of guilt … …

… … {about 5-10 seconds of silence} …

… … I forgive myself for slipping back into anorexia … … because I am now truly ready to end the past … …

… … {about 5-10 seconds of silence} …

… … I forgive myself for slipping back into anorexia … … because I am now truly ready to look and move forward … …

… … {about 5-10 seconds of silence} …

… … I forgive myself for slipping back into anorexia … … because I am now truly ready to accept myself fully … …

… … {about 5-10 seconds of silence} …

… … I forgive myself for slipping back into anorexia … … because I am now truly ready to be myself … …

… … {about 5-10 seconds of silence} …

+++ End of Version 2 +++

… … I save my life, in love and gratitude towards myself … … with the certainty that I want it exactly this way … …

… … {about 5-10 seconds of silence} …

… … I save my life, in love and gratitude towards myself … … with the certainty that I can truly do it exactly this way … …

… … {about 5-10 seconds of silence} …

… … I save my life, in love and gratitude towards myself … … with the certainty that I am truly worth being loved … …

… … {about 5-10 seconds of silence} …

... ... I save my life, in love and gratitude towards myself ...
... with the certainty that self-love is forever within me ... ...

... ... {about 5-10 seconds of silence} ...

... ... I save my life, in love and gratitude towards myself ...
... with the certainty that my self-love is real and honest ... ...

... ... {about 5-10 seconds of silence} ...

All Titles in the Series

Volume 1: Smoking Cessation
Volume 2: Anxiety and Restlessness
Volume 3: Burnout
Volume 4: Reducing Overweight
Volume 5: Coping with the Past
Volume 6: Suicidal Thoughts and Attempts
Volume 7: Psycho-Oncology
Volume 8: Obsessions and Tics
Volume 9: Self-Confidence and Decision-Making
Volume 10: Grief Work
Volume 11: Psychosomatics
Volume 12: Chronic Pain
Volume 13: Depressive Thoughts
Volume 14: Panic Attacks
Volume 15: Domestic Violence, Victim Support
Volume 16: Post-Traumatic Stress
Volume 17: Exam Anxiety and Stage Fright
Volume 18: Anti-Violence Training, Offender Support
Volume 19: Addiction Tendencies
Volume 20: Social Phobia and Fear of Contact
Volume 21: Nail Biting
Volume 22: Self-Awareness and Self-Love
Volume 23: Teeth Grinding and Night Clenching
Volume 24: Feelings of Guilt
Volume 25: Fear in Crowds
Volume 26: Fear of Flying, Aviophobia
Volume 27: Fear in Enclosed Spaces, Claustrophobia
Volume 28: Tinnitus, Ear Noises
Volume 29: Fear of Heights
Volume 30: Neurodermatitis

Volume 31: Finding Inner Balance
Volume 32: Overcoming Loneliness
Volume 33: Fear of Illness, Hypochondria
Volume 34: Anticipatory Anxiety, Fear of Fear
Volume 35: Jealousy in Relationships
Volume 36: Driving Anxiety
Volume 37: New Start after Separation
Volume 38: Fear of Injections
Volume 39: Heart Anxiety Neurosis
Volume 40: Overcoming Resentment and Anger
Volume 41: Resolving Blockages and Positive Thinking
Volume 42: Stress Reduction, Stress Management
Volume 43: Body Relaxation
Volume 44: Deep Relaxation
Volume 45: Fear of the Dark
Volume 46: Falling Asleep and Staying Asleep
Volume 47: Compulsive Buying
Volume 48: Restless Legs Syndrome
Volume 49: Bulimia
Volume 50: Anorexia
Volume 51: Overcoming Nightmares
Volume 52: Imagined Deformity
Volume 53: Overcoming Distrust, Finding Trust
Volume 54: Processing Failures
Volume 55: Humiliation, Emotional Hurt
Volume 56: Distressing Compassion, Vicarious Suffering
Volume 57: Self-Forgiveness
Volume 58: Self-Awareness, Self-Confidence
Volume 59: Saying No
Volume 60: Assertiveness
Volume 61: Setting Boundaries and Self-Assertion
Volume 62: Decision-Making Ability

Volume 63: Success Orientation
Volume 64: Ruminating, Circular Thinking
Volume 65: Accepting Pregnancy
Volume 66: Birth Preparation
Volume 67: Spiritual Opening
Volume 68: Joy of Life and Inner Lightness
Volume 69: Patience and Inner Peace
Volume 70: Fibromyalgia and Rheumatism
Volume 71: Irritable Bowel Syndrome, Crohn's Disease
Volume 72: Fear of Nausea, Emetophobia
Volume 73: Stuttering and Cluttering, Speech Flow Disorders
Volume 74: Concentration and Knowledge Anchoring
Volume 75: Vitality and Spontaneity
Volume 76: Searching for Meaning and Finding Goals
Volume 77: Life Crises, Life Events
Volume 78: Workaholism, Goal Obsession
Volume 79: Helper Syndrome, Helpless Helpers
Volume 80: Medication Abuse
Volume 81: Gambling Addiction
Volume 82: Internet Addiction, Smartphone Addiction
Volume 83: Hoarding Disorder, Compulsive Collecting
Volume 84: Conspiracy Thoughts, Overvalued Ideas
Volume 85: Fear of Operations and Treatments
Volume 86: Fear of Aging
Volume 87: Travel Anxiety
Volume 88: Anxiety When Urinating, Paruresis
Volume 89: Fear of Intimacy and Togetherness
Volume 90: Fear of Blushing
Volume 91: Coming Out in Homosexuality
Volume 92: Charisma Training
Volume 93: Migraines and Chronic Headaches
Volume 94: Overcoming Allergies, Bronchial Asthma

Volume 95: Normalizing Blood Pressure
Volume 96: Compulsive Perfectionism
Volume 97: Sports Hypnosis, Motivation
Volume 98: Sports Hypnosis, Performance Enhancement
Volume 99: Determination and Focus
Volume 100: Encountering the Inner Child
Volume 101: Cravings, Binge Eating
Volume 102: Stimulating Metabolism
Volume 103: Bipolar Mood Swings
Volume 104: Borderline, Identity Crises
Volume 105: Hypomania, Euphoria, Mania
Volume 106: Restlessness, Agitation
Volume 107: Nervous Breakdown
Volume 108: Adjustment Disorders
Volume 109: Self-Alienation, Depersonalization
Volume 110: Ending Self-Pity
Volume 111: Primary Gain of Illness
Volume 112: Secondary Gain of Illness
Volume 113: Bullying, Victim Support
Volume 114: Letting Go of Envy and Jealousy
Volume 115: Fear of Spiders, Arachnophobia
Volume 116: Fear of Dogs or Cats
Volume 117: Fear of Strangers, Xenophobia
Volume 118: Excessive Worries, Generalized Anxiety
Volume 119: Strengthening Sense of Responsibility
Volume 120: Unrequited Love, Heartache
Volume 121: Work-Life Balance
Volume 122: Letting Go of Unattainable Goals
Volume 123: Allowing and Accepting Help
Volume 124: Letting Go of Adult Children
Volume 125: Tourette Syndrome
Volume 126: Life Changes and New Starts

Volume 127: Accepting Life in a Wheelchair
Volume 128: Understanding and Overcoming Homesickness
Volume 129: Understanding and Overcoming Wanderlust
Volume 130: Dizziness, Meniere's Disease
Volume 131: Overcoming Aggression
Volume 132: Cutting and Self-Harm
Volume 133: Hair Pulling, Trichotillomania
Volume 134: Postpartum Depression
Volume 135: For Relatives of Dementia Patients
Volume 136: Self-Harm, Artificial Disorders
Volume 137: Activating Self-Healing Powers
Volume 138: Preventing Depression Relapse
Volume 139: Reactive Psychoses, Follow-Up
Volume 140: Obsessive Thoughts and Impulses
Volume 141: Compulsive Checking
Volume 142: Compulsive Counting, Symmetry Obsession
Volume 143: Compulsive Washing, Cleanliness Obsession
Volume 144: Compulsive Questioning
Volume 145: Dissociative Paralysis
Volume 146: Phantom Pain
Volume 147: Overcoming Complaining
Volume 148: Hay Fever, Pollen Allergy
Volume 149: Sexual Abuse, Victim Support
Volume 150: Standing Strong Against Sexism, #metoo
Volume 151: Binge Eating
Volume 152: Overcoming Thoughts of Revenge
Volume 153: Detachment from the Aggressor, Stockholm Syndrome
Volume 154: Courage to Separate
Volume 155: Chronic Fatigue, Exhaustion
Volume 156: Fear of the Future, Existential Anxiety
Volume 157: Excessive Worry About Children
Volume 158: Fear of Failure

Volume 159: Ending Distrust and Control
Volume 160: Dejection, Dysphoria
Volume 161: Boreout, Chronic Boredom
Volume 162: Bipolar Disorders, Relapse Prevention
Volume 163: Mania, Relapse Prevention
Volume 164: Nihilism, Feelings of Worthlessness
Volume 165: Thumb Sucking
Volume 166: Being Brave
Volume 167: Being Proud
Volume 168: Overcoming Shyness
Volume 169: Being Able to Delegate Responsibility
Volume 170: Being Able to Show Emotions
Volume 171: Letting Go of Guilt, Victim Support
Volume 172: Processing Guilt, Offender Support
Volume 173: Mood Swings, Cyclothymia
Volume 174: Lack of Drive, Vital Sadness
Volume 175: Hearing Voices with Reality Reference
Volume 176: Confident Communication
Volume 177: Standing Up for Oneself
Volume 178: Taking New Paths
Volume 179: Confident Job Application
Volume 180: No Longer Being Taken Advantage Of
Volume 181: End of Submissiveness
Volume 182: Depressive Numbness
Volume 183: Mood Drops, Affective Incontinence
Volume 184: Mood Instability
Volume 185: Somatoform Disorders
Volume 186: Stomach Ulcer, Psychosomatic
Volume 187: Accepting Amputation
Volume 188: Overcoming and Letting Go of Hatred
Volume 189: Ending Accusations
Volume 190: Allowing Tears, Being Able to Cry

Volume 191: Finding and Sorting Repressed Feelings
Volume 192: Somatoform Pain
Volume 193: Living Autonomously
Volume 194: Anhedonia, Joylessness
Volume 195: Persistent Sadness
Volume 196: Obesity, Food Addiction
Volume 197: Parents of Abused Children
Volume 198: Letting Go and Letting Be
Volume 199: Childhood Sexual Abuse
Volume 200: Fear of Loss

www.ingramcontent.com/pod-product-compliance
Lightning Source LLC
Chambersburg PA
CBHW030452220526
45464CB00006B/2508